the content within this book without the consent of the author or copyright owner. Legal action will be pursued if this is breached.

<u>Disclaimer Notice:</u>

Please note the information contained within this document is for educational and entertainment purposes only. Every attempt has been made to provide accurate, up to date and reliable complete information. No warranties of any kind are expressed or implied. Readers acknowledge that the author is not engaging in the rendering of legal, financial, medical or professional advice.

By reading this document, the reader agrees that under no circumstances are we responsible for any losses, direct or indirect, which are incurred as a result of the use of information contained within this document, including, but not limited to, —errors, omissions, or inaccuracies.

TABLE OF CONTENTS

Introduction

You visit the doctor regularly to maintain your health. That's certainly smart. Before your next appointment, however, consider this: when was the last time your doctor asked about your diet?

Although physicians are perfectly aware of the connection between our health and the food we put into our body, this is a question they rarely, if ever, pose. They appear to be more interested in prescribing medications than treating and preventing health problems in a more natural and effective way. This is especially disconcerting as more and more people suffer from wheat sensitivity, allergy, or celiac disease.

The problem with wheat is caused by gluten, one of the proteins found in modern-day wheat. It can damage the smaller intestine and make digesting wheat difficult or impossible. It can cause fatigue, nausea, diarrhea and other, more serious discomforts, such as damaging the small intestine. Celiac disease is serious, and physicians need to start paying attention.

Processed wheat, which is found everywhere, isn't healthy for anyone. For people with celiac disease, it can be a daily nightmare. That is why going gluten-free is becoming increasingly popular. People are learning the effects of modern wheat and are starting to take control of their own health.

For people who are sensitive or allergic to wheat, going gluten-free can be life-changing. It can help them rid the body of irritating toxins and help them function normally again.

For others, who are not gluten-sensitive, abstaining from gluten is a way of eating healthier, feeling better, and having more energy.

Food matters. What we consume is critical to our health. The fact is, gluten adds little to our lives but can cause considerable damage. Going gluten-free is a return to eating in a way that promotes optimum health and wellbeing. For anyone who believes that we have been eating wheat for thousands of years without a problem, you will soon learn why that is incorrect.

Even for those who are not suffering from celiac disease or wheat sensitivity, a gluten-free diet can be a prevention against disease. Gluten is known to cause serious inflammations, and inflammations can increase the risk of arthritis and coronary diseases. Using food to prevent the onset of these problems enables us to enjoy a healthier lifestyle. This makes far more sense than treating diseases with medications that can have harmful side effects.

Gluten is all around us, which can make going gluten-free quite a challenge. With so many food items made of wheat, barley, or rye, all of which contain gluten, and with more food products containing hidden wheat, the idea of eating gluten-free may seem like deprivation. Quite the contrary. You can still eat the cookies, cakes, and pasta you love. You will simply be preparing them differently.

If you are suffering from celiac disease, going gluten-free is a must. But other intestinal issues, such as diarrhea and irritable bowel syndrome have also been relieved with a gluten-free diet. Researchers are linking more and more gastrointestinal problems to gluten.

In addition, we'll take a look at the surprising connection between gluten-free, ADHD, and autism.

You will soon discover the options available to you, and how to make gluten-free eating a part of your healthy lifestyle.

1

WHEAT AND CELIAC

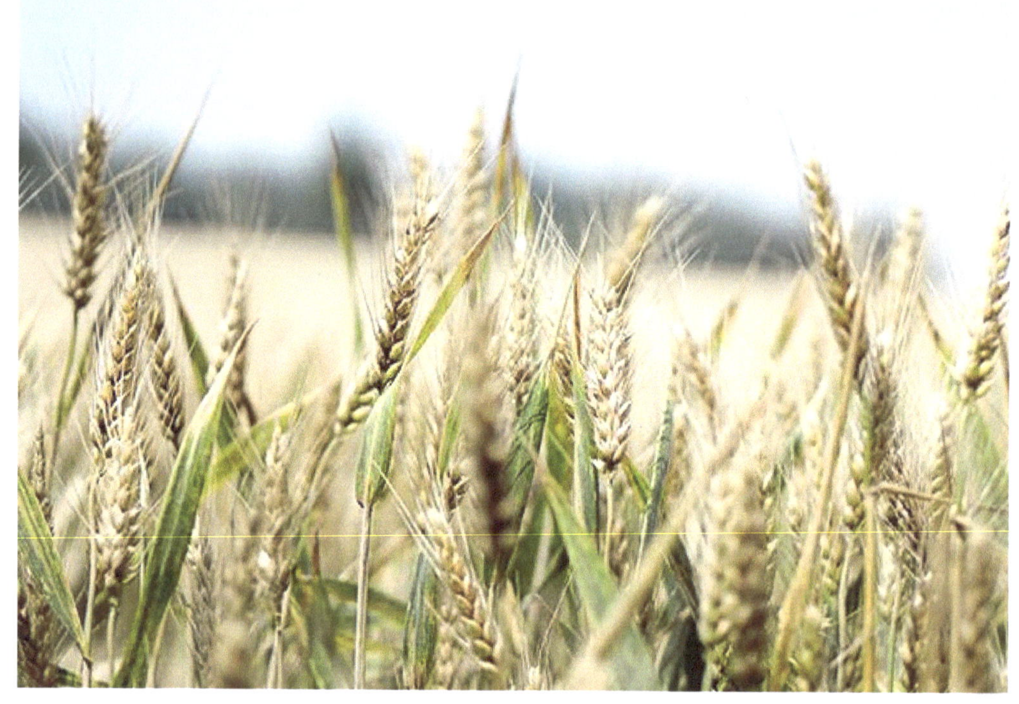

Chapter 1
Wheat and Celiac Disease – The Downside of Gluten

Wheat has been around for thousands of years. It's easy to grow and quite nutritious. It was probably one of the first food items our forefathers gathered to feed themselves. Wheat was truly life-giving.

For all these thousands of years, the whole grain kernel was ground and used to bake bread or prepare cereals. Fresh, whole grain has always been a part of our diet without being harmful to our health.

It's not until the 1960s and 70s that people began to realize that the wheat they are consuming is making them sick.

What happened? Have our bodies changed? No. It's the wheat we have relied on for thousands of years that has been changed and twisted into something our forefathers wouldn't recognize.

Industrialization has been good to mankind, but it hasn't always been kind to the food we consume.

Let's start with white flour, the first food that we would call "processed." In 1870, the steel roller mill allowed wheat to be separated to refine the wheat into a white powder. "White" flour was considered fancy.

So, to meet consumer demand, white flour was produced en masse, and the rest of the kernel, the nutritious part, was tossed aside. Within 10 years, all flour was white and seriously lacking in nutrients. Ten years was all the time it took to change thousands of years of nourishment into something "fancy" and lacking in many nutrients.

That was only the beginning, however. By the 1950s, technology once again let us "improve" our wheat. New techniques allowed for genetically-altered seeds, fertilizers, and harmful pesticides to increase wheat production. Again, everyone rejoiced. More wheat for everyone! Cake for one and all!

While the production of wheat increased, its nutritional value was being mangled into something unrecognizable. At the same time, inflammations and immune diseases were being linked directly to this new, "improved" wheat.

Anyone who believes that gluten-free is just a modern phase is half-right. It is indeed something new and modern. But it is not a phase. An increasing number of people are suffering from the effects of modern wheat and refined flour.

The degree can vary – from a bit of wheat sensitivity to greater intolerance to celiac disease, which is the inability to process any amount of wheat due to problems in the small intestines. Especially in the case of celiac disease, the digestive system views gluten as invaders and reacts accordingly. As it tries to attack these toxins, the lining of the gut itself can become damaged, resulting in leaks, inflammation, and other problems. Serious gastrointestinal problems are the result.

The number of people diagnosed with celiac disease has quadrupled in the past 50 years. One percent of the population suffers from celiac disease, and the number is rising. Wheat sensitivity affects up to 8 percent of the population. It is obvious that new "improved" wheat is making people sick.

In studies comparing modern, "improved" wheat to old wheat (called Einkorn), it was found that the old wheat had no harmful effects at all. No one who consumed unrefined wheat suffered any ill side effects or gastrointestinal problems. The same studies showed that modern wheat can affect our autoimmune system in harmful ways, leading to celiac disease and allergies.

People who are not allergic to modern wheat can still suffer. A 2013 study had healthy participants eat either new or old wheat for two months. The group that consumed the old wheat found their cholesterol level had decreased and their level of potassium and magnesium had increased. The opposite was true of the group given new wheat.

It is important to distinguish between gluten sensitivity and celiac disease, although they can have the same symptoms. Gluten sensitivity results in feelings of fatigue, bloating, diarrhea, nausea, and headaches. Many people don't even associate those feeling with wheat, so it's critical that doctors ask the right questions and test for wheat allergy.

People diagnosed with celiac disease suffer from identical symptoms, but the problem is more specifically defined. The gluten attacks the inflammatory system and can damage the small intestine. Inflammation is linked with a myriad of problems, such as heart disease, Alzheimer's, diabetes, and others.

The role of gluten itself is still being studied. What is clear, however, is that this modern, improved wheat is causing some serious illness. While wheat can be found almost everywhere, it is most commonly used in breads, cakes, cookies, pasta, creamed soups, sauces, cereal, and some salad dressings.

Rye wheat can be found in rye breads, beer, and some cereals.

Of course, wheat can be found in many other hidden places, and we will discuss this in much greater detail.

What is clear is that people who have eliminated wheat and gluten from their diet feel better and become healthier. With anyone suffering from celiac disease going gluten-free is a necessity. For others, it is a choice in an effort to enjoy increased health.

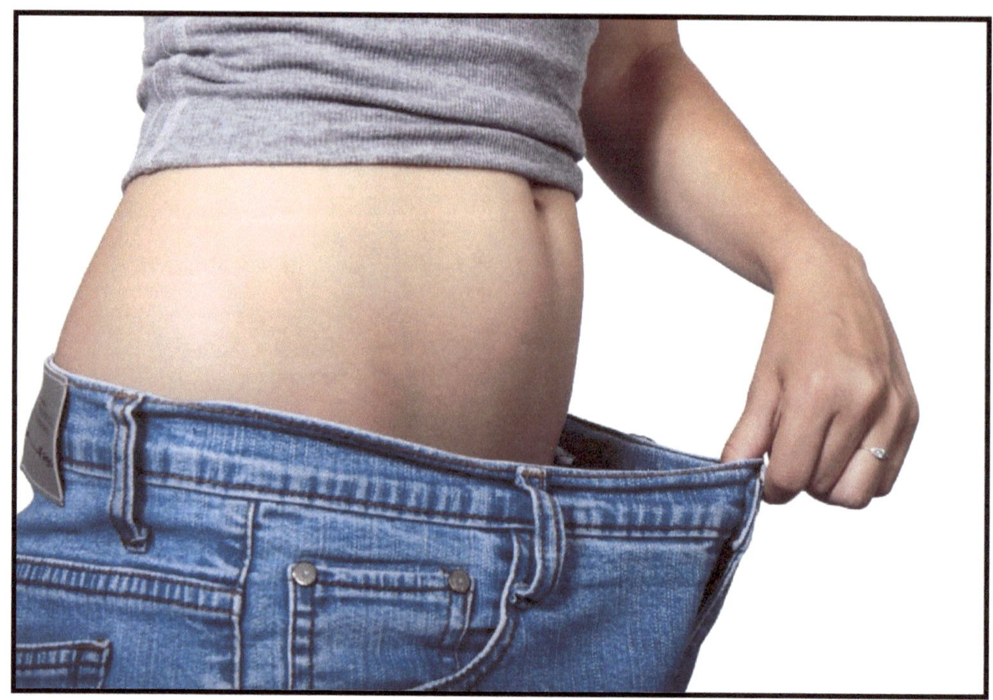

Most people also chose a gluten-free diet in order to lose weight. A diet filled with breads, cakes, and noodles is high in carbohydrates and will very likely pack on the pounds. The reason for that is that refined wheat can cause a sugar spike. That means you use sugar for fuel while fat just gets stored and piled up. People find losing weight by cutting refined flour to be much easier and quicker.

Celiac disease can run in families and can be hereditary. People with parents or grandparents who have suffered from celiac disease have a 1 in 10 chance of becoming grain-intolerant.

CHAPTER 2

SHOPPING GLUTEN-FREE

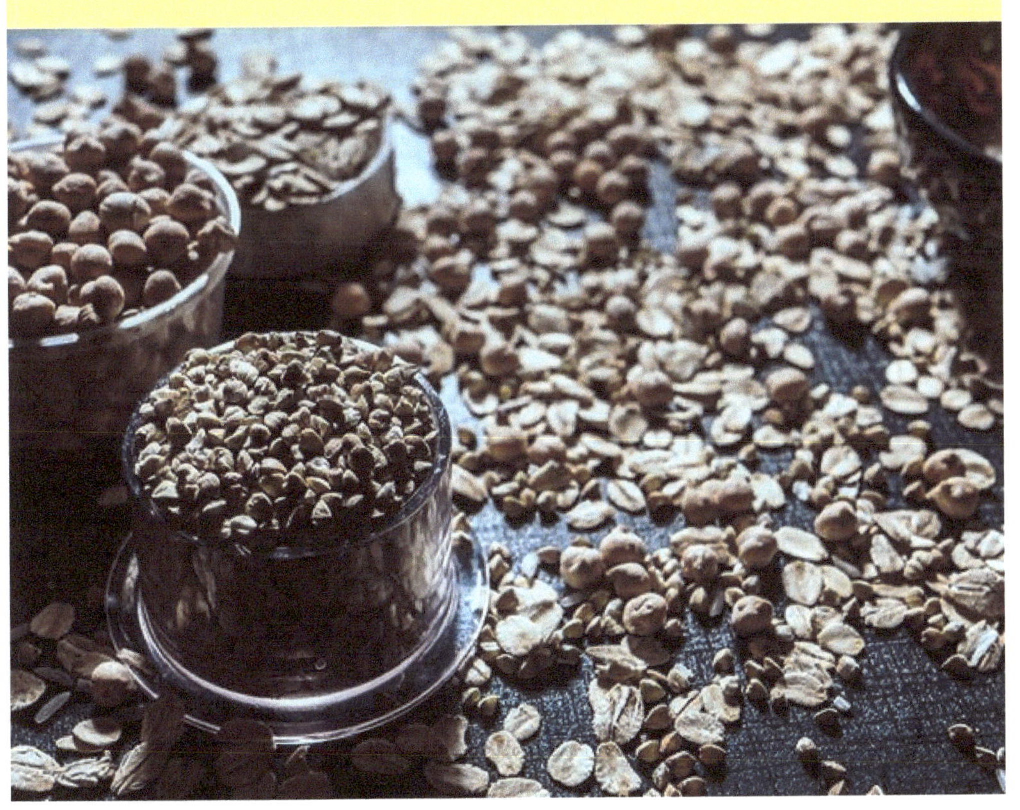

Chapter 2

Shopping Gluten-Free

When you begin to shop gluten-free, it can be a bit confusing and overwhelming. You might panic about missing out on your favorite meals. It may seem that there is nothing for you to eat. You'll quickly find, however, that is not the case. You won't miss anything.

Finding delicious foods that are gluten-free is easier than you think. You are likely to find a few tasty food options that you haven't considered. Once you know what to watch out for, you'll master the supermarket aisle like a gluten pro.

Besides, if one or more member of your family is gluten-intolerant while the rest are able to eat wheat, don't prepare separate meals. Gluten-free meals are NOT a punishment, and anyone suffering from celiac disease or gluten intolerance should not be made to feel guilty or different. Omitting gluten from your diet is eating healthy, and that is something your entire family should be doing.

Have a Plan

Your trip to the market starts with a list. Walking up and down the aisles can lead to serious temptations. Supermarkets are deliberately designed to tempt you and lure you into buying things you don't need. You don't want to roam randomly. Before you leave the house, before you even create your shopping list, plan your meals.

Don't approach meal-planning negatively, as in, "Oh, I can't eat pasta … bread … cookies." Eating gluten-free is not about subtracting and deprivation. It's all about eating better. Plan the meals you enjoy and think in terms of substitutions. How can you improve this recipe? For example, if you want to prepare pasta, do so. Simply plan on using zoodles (zucchini noodles) or gluten-free pasta in your preparation.

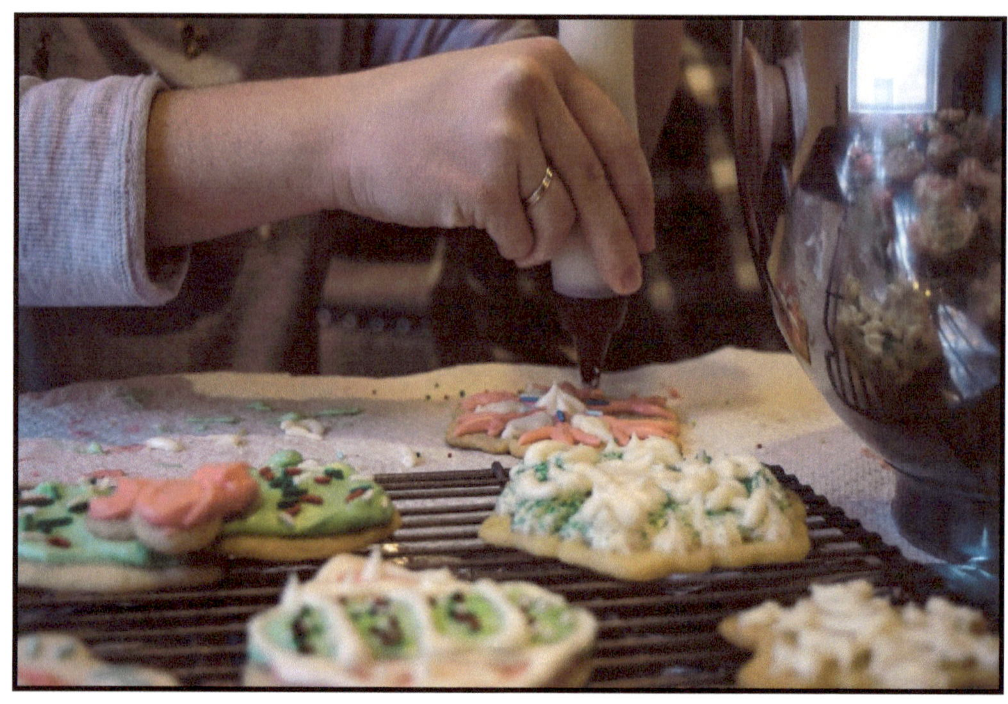

Feel like baking some cookies for the kids? All you need to do is substitute wheat-free flour in your recipe. We'll discuss substitution later in this book. One or two gluten-free cookbooks will provide you with inspiration and help you understand how delicious gluten-free meals can be. They are an excellent investment.

Think in terms of variety. The greater the variety of food you eat, the more nutrition you consume. And don't forget about herbs and spices, most of which are quite nutrient-packed. Shopping gluten-free will expand your food world.

There are many places to purchase gluten-free products. (Aren't you lucky!). There are the around-every-corner supermarkets, specialty stores, health food stores, outdoor farmer markets, and online. By all means, make yourself available to all of these options. However, make the supermarket your main shopping place. There are reasons for that.

First, gluten-free is catching on, and most markets now carry gluten-free products or have an entire gluten-free aisle. The deli section is likely to offer a number of gluten-free items. By shopping at the regular market, you won't feel that you are shopping "differently," and that is psychologically important. You're not different, you're just smart.

Any farmer's market, of course, is a treasure trove of healthy produce, so you definitely want to be there whenever possible. As for specialty health food stores and online shopping, keep that in reserve as a valuable last resort for any product you can't find in stores.

Now that you've planed your meals, you are ready to create your shopping list. Keep in mind that prepared and pre-packaged foods frequently have hidden sugars and gluten. If you are unsure, contact the manufacturer for more details. In addition to bringing your shopping list, you should also have a gluten-free food/ingredient list for interpreting difficult labels.

We recommend that if possible, you shop without young children, whose sticky little fingers invariably reach for chocolate, cookies, and other snacks with abandon. You need to maintain control of the shopping situation.

You at the Supermarket

Okay, you are at the supermarket, wheeling that shopping cart down the aisle. Now, what?

All supermarkets tend to be laid out in the same way, so it's easy to avoid "dangerous" aisles and sections. When shopping gluten-free, you'll be spending most of your time circling the perimeter of the store, and not the aisles.

The produce section is usually near the entrance, so that's where you want to head first. Stock up on fresh, in-season fruits and vegetables. This is a chance to pick up produce you haven't tried before and broaden your food selection. Salads are always healthy, tasty, and gluten-free, but take care with croutons and dressing.

The bread aisle can be tricky and tempting. You need to forego most bread offerings and look for gluten-free bread. However, even here you need to be careful. Anything labeled "gluten-free" may be filled with additional fats and sugars. In addition to studying labels carefully, make a note of the expiration date. Gluten-free breads usually have fewer preservatives and may expire more quickly.

You've made it to the deli. You feel pretty safe here, as cheeses don't contain gluten. Technically, they don't, but many low-fat cheeses may contain fillers that are wheat-based. As for cold-cut, they are likely to contain wheat-based fillers. More about that later, but ask the person behind the counter before making any purchases.

You should be able to make good use of the bulk food section. The good news is there are many types of gluten-free, wheat-free flours from which to choose. Gluten-free flours can function and taste differently from regular flours, so you should become familiar with how these flours are best used. A gluten-free cookbook can be very helpful in helping you create the delicious desserts you thought you'd never enjoy again.

Some of the most popular, gluten-free, wheat-free flours are as follows:

1. Coconut flour – a great baking flour
2. Corn flour – made from corn and used in baking and coating.
3. Oat flour – when made of natural oats, oat flour is gluten-free. Great for cookies and baking.
4. Brown rice flour – this is easy to digest. In addition, pasta made with brown rice flour is your best alternative to the standard white-flour pasta. There is white rice flour, as well, which is gluten-free. However, the white type of rice flour has been polished of most of its vitamins B and important minerals. It won't harm you, but you won't get the same nutrition that you would with brown rice flour.
5. Almond flour – made from healthy nuts. Almond flour can be used in almost any kind of baking.
6. Tapioca flour – this isn't really a baking/cooking flour. It is frequently used as a thickener for sauces and to create a roux.
7. Chickpea flour – this healthy flour contains needed fiber and minerals. It is best used for pancakes and waffles.
8. Sorghum flour – this is a heavy flour. When used in baking, it is frequently combined with tapioca flour.

9. Cassava flour – this flour contains few nutrients other than vitamin C, but it can easily be used for baking.

10. Amaranth Flour – this is a nutrient-packed flour that, like sorghum, can be mixed with another flour for baking.

11. Buckwheat flour actually isn't a flour, but a very healthful seed. Great for making pancakes.

12. Teff flour – another flour that can be used with other gluten-free flours for baking.

13. Cricket flour – this is actually made from roasted crickets, but don't let that keep you from trying it. It's nutrient-dense and has a nutty flavor.

14. All-purpose gluten-free flour – this is made from a combination of the above flours and can be used for all-purpose baking.

As you can see, gluten-free cooking offers you lots of choices, and you should experiment to see which flour works best for you. Flours made from coconut or almond can lend a delightful flavor to your baked goods.

A word of caution: When flours are displayed in bulk, there can be some cross-contamination when a customer uses the same scooper to bag glutenous and non-gluten types of flours. If that is a serious concern, get your gluten-free flour from a market or a health food store that has a separate gluten-free section, or order through the internet.

You and your cart, which is getting pretty full, have made it to the dairy section. Notice that you are still wandering the perimeter of the market instead of roaming the aisles.

Milk and dairy do not contain gluten, but be careful of additives. Yogurts and ice cream can contain all types of flavoring, so read the labels carefully. And, as previously stated, any item labeled "diet" or "low fat" is likely to contain gluten fillers.

If you're in search of snacks, you are likely to end up in one of the aisles. Check ingredient labels carefully. As an alternative, prepare your own tasty snack by mixing gluten-free granola with chopped nuts or dried fruits.

When you arrive at the meat and fish section, you are in a gluten-free zone, except for the prepared and coated meats, which you will ignore. Focus on lean meats and fish to prepare tasty and healthy meals.

GETTING STARTED WITH THE GLUTEN-FREE LIFE

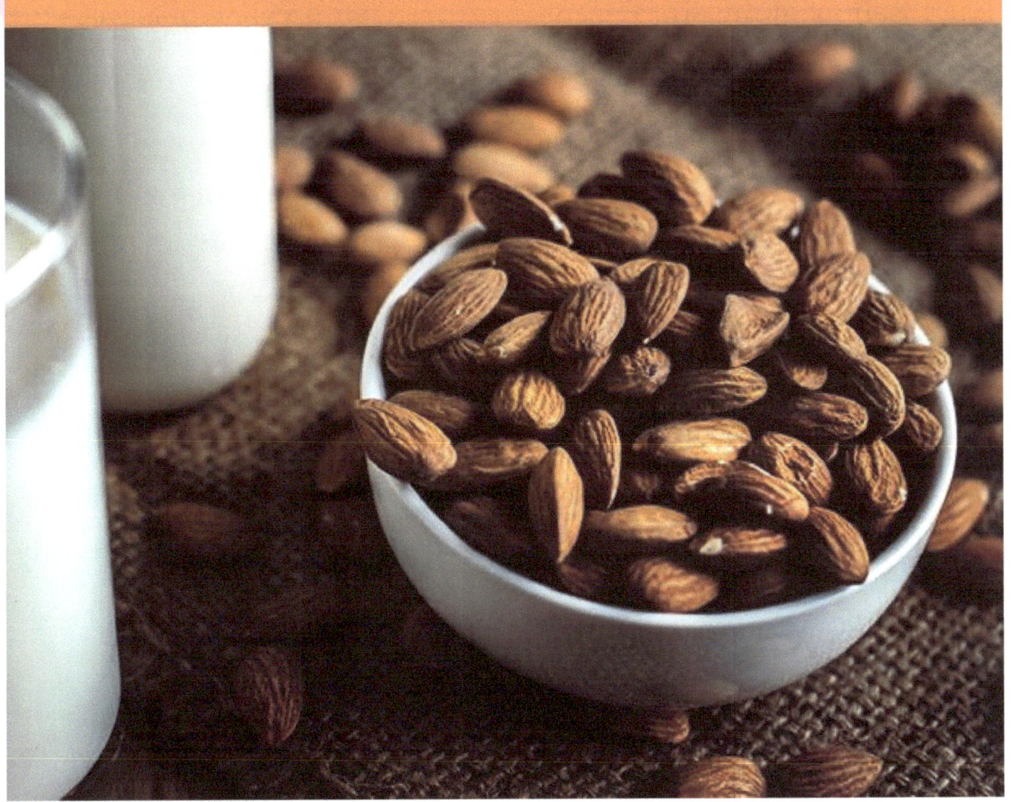

Chapter 3

Getting Started with the Gluten-Free Life

If you are thinking about going gluten-free in order to live more healthfully, good for you. It's an excellent decision. If you have been diagnosed as gluten-intolerant, or worse, with celiac disease, you may feel frustrated and overwhelmed. Where on earth do you even start? You have a right to be concerned, because your health is at stake. Going gluten-free is a must for you. It's up to you to make the experience as enjoyable as possible.

Your first step is to become as informed as you can, and the purpose of this book is to help you get started. This is just the beginning, however. Talk to a doctor who is knowledgeable and proactive when it comes to diets and health; i.e., a doctor who doesn't simply write out prescriptions.

Meet with a trained nutritionist who is familiar with celiac disease. He or she can provide a great deal of detailed information regarding *your* specific situation and help you plan healthful meals for you and your family. Then check out celiac support groups in your area. Members have experienced the same frustrations you are now going through and will understand.

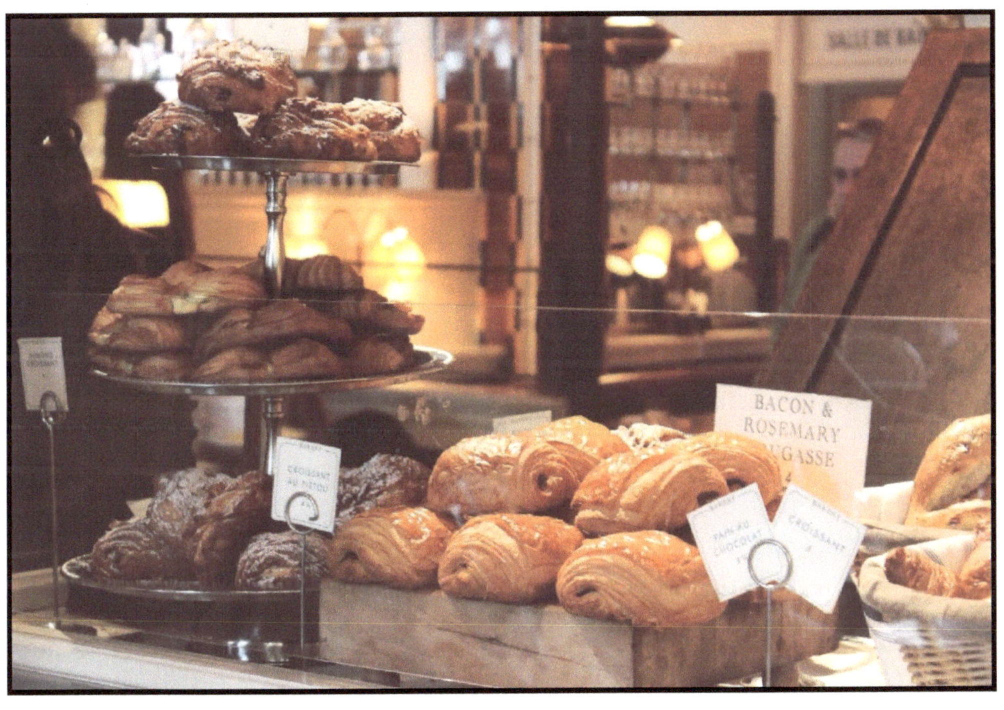

You also need to become product-savvy. Wheat can hide in the most unexpected places, especially in prepared foods. Read labels, and if you have any questions, call the company and ask for specifics about the ingredients. You have every right to know what goes into your body.

A Gluten-Free Kitchen

Once you know what foods to bring into the house (keep in mind fresh is always best), you need to prepare your kitchen in order to avoid cross-contamination.

We have already mentioned that it is best for the entire family to enjoy gluten-free cooking instead of you preparing a separate meal. In the event you don't do that, you need to dedicate special household products to your gluten-free cooking. That includes pots, pans, cutting board, and utensils. Clean out the toaster to remove wheat crumbs. Gluten can attach itself to these items and cause cross-contamination.

Start your gluten-free journey from scratch. If the entire family is involved, as they should be, toss out any gluten-containing food items from the freezer, refrigerator and cupboards and replace them with gluten-free equivalents. It may seem overwhelming to toss your favorite bagel, pasta, and cookies, but once you learn how to prepare gluten-free alternatives, you won't miss them. There is every chance you will actual prefer the tasty gluten-free meals and snacks.

If other family members remain on a gluten-filled diet, place their food in a separate, dedicated area. After preparing their meals, be sure to thoroughly clean any affected surfaces.

Cleaning Out the Bathroom

For anyone starting out on the gluten-free life, it may come as a surprise that the kitchen isn't the only room in the house filled with potential dangers.

Your bathroom may be stocked with gluten that can negatively affect your gluten intolerance. Many ordinary cosmetics and hygiene items contain wheat. As a matter of fact, wheat is a favorite exfoliant for the face and body and can be found in any number of lotions and cleansers.

Read the labels on the following bathroom products carefully:

- Soaps and gels
- Facial scrubs
- Shampoo
- Skin lotions
- Toothpaste
- Lipstick
- Hairspray

Many of these products call themselves "natural" or "organic" due to the wheat content. If you need to replace any product, look for products containing shea butter or oils such as coconuts or jojoba oil, which are excellent moisturizers.

Luckily, there are a number of cosmetic lines that specialize in gluten-free products. Check the internet for specifics.

In addition, if you are wheat-intolerant, beware of kissing someone wearing lipstick that may contain wheat. Rule of thumb: if you know someone well enough to kiss, you should know them well enough to explain your wheat-intolerance and have them check their cosmetics.

You and Booze

The good news is, you don't have to give up alcohol to enjoy a gluten-free life. You do need to beware of beer, distilled products, and any malt beverages.

You can, however, enjoy bourbon, gin, tequila, rum, cognacs, vodka, and wine.

Gluten and Your Medicine Cabinet

While there is no cure for celiac disease, you may be taking medications for other issues. While you can discuss medications with your doctor, physicians aren't always informed about specific medicines and their ingredients. Your best bet is to talk to the pharmacist and explain your situation. It is always better to be informed and cautious.

A number of pharmaceuticals contain starch from corn, potato and wheat. Laws regarding labeling pharmaceuticals can be hazy. Companies are not required to list the type of starch they use. Best to err on the side of caution, as the wrong medication may cause abdominal problems, diarrhea and other symptoms. You don't want your pharmaceuticals to make you sick!

If you have any doubts about the medication you are taking, have the pharmacist call the manufacturer, or call the company yourself. You are entitled to know how their products are manufactured.

While you're with your helpful pharmacist, ask him or her about supplements and vitamins. Since celiac disease makes absorption of nutrients difficult (more about that in another chapter of this book), you should be taking supplements to make up for the loss and help alleviate nutrient deficiency.

Gluten-Free Pantry

When you're eating gluten-free, it's important to have a well-stocked pantry. Otherwise, unexpected guests or coming home hungry and wanting dinner now, or simple, human cravings can have you throwing up your hands in despair. "Fine, we'll order in pizza!"

If you don't want that to happen, you need to be prepared with a well-stocked pantry. You should have all the ingredients for a delicious, gluten-free meal on hand whenever needed.

All of us turn to food for comfort at times. That's fine, as long as the comfort is healthful and nourishing.

For a quick breakfast when you are in a hurry, keep a container of gluten-free buckwheat on hand. Try it with a poached egg to get your going in the morning.

Have gluten-free breads on hand for a satisfying sandwich at lunch.

For a tasty dinner, make sure you have plenty of gluten-free flours, brown rice, gluten-free corn tortillas to prepare meal and vegetable dishes. Check out gluten-free pastas online.

Snacks can be tough. When kids come home from school and bring their friends, you need a plan. Be prepared to serve up popcorn, gluten-free crackers and cheese, trail mix, or banana slices with peanut butter at a moment's notice.

Necessary Foods in Your Pantry

In addition to fresh produce and lean meats and fish, there are certain items that should always be on your shelves. You will note that many of them are for seasoning and elevating a dish when cooking. You really should never be without:

- Garlic
- Rice, quinoa and potatoes
- Many different types of gluten-free flours
- A high-quality olive oil and other oils, such as coconut oil.
- A few high-quality vinegars
- A variety of lentils and bean, preferably the dry kind
- A variety of broths, such as beef, chicken, and fish broths, preferably homemade
- A variety of nuts and seeds
- Mustard
- A variety of spices to liven up your dishes
- Fresh herbs
- Tamari sauce (a gluten-free soy sauce)
- Sour cream
- Parmesan cheese
- Eggs
- Yogurts (read labels prior to purchasing)

- Cans of tuna fish

- Dried mushrooms

- Canned tomatoes (check label)

- Fire-roasted tomatoes and chilis for added heat

There are many other foods that can make it into your kitchen, but these essentials should enable you to prepare a healthful, gluten-free meal at any time.

CHAPTER 4

DINING OUT AND BEING SOCIAL

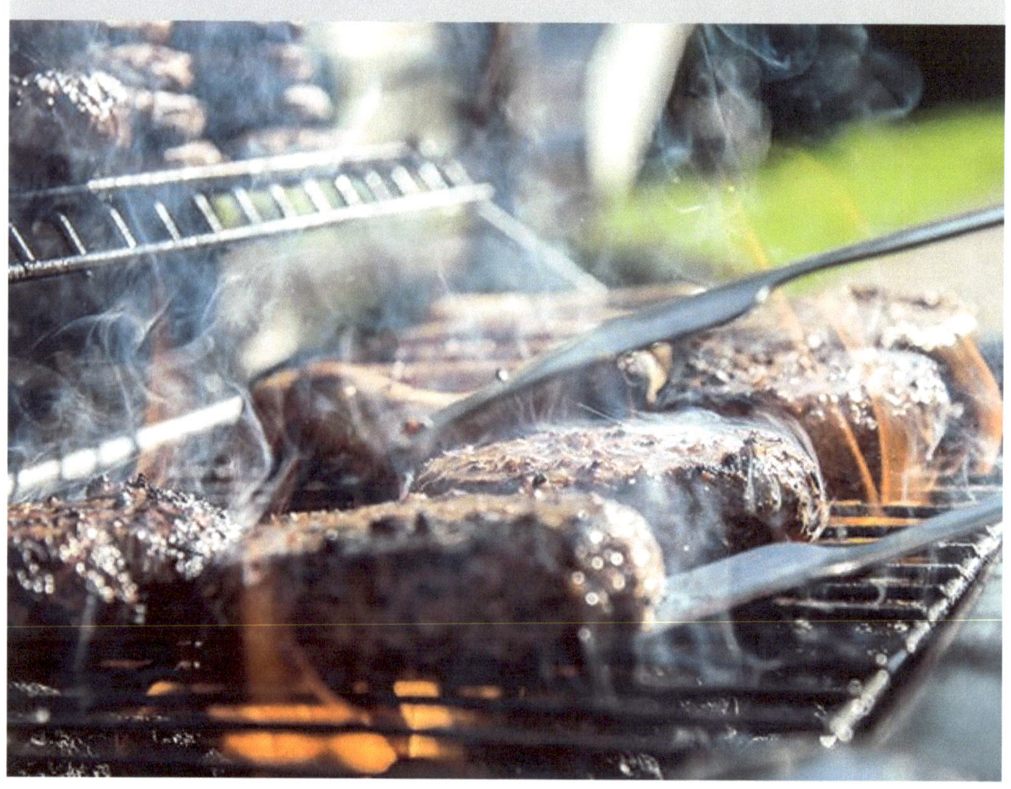

Chapter 4

Dining Out and Being Social

At times, it might feel as if changing your eating habits to remove gluten from your life is the worst thing that can happen. But then, as you discover a world of healthy alternatives and begin to eat foods you've never even considered, you relax and enjoy all the benefits.

There is one aspect of going gluten-free, however, that can unnerve even experienced old-timers. Eating someplace that isn't home. Handling eating out, either on your own or with friends, can feel overwhelming. And how do you handle dinner invitations? The fact is, other people may not understand what you are going through.

Unless you want to turn into a hermit, however, you are going to have to socialize. We are social beings, and we need to be around other people.

This book will help you overcome the challenges of eating out and turn you into a worry-free social butterfly.

First, you shouldn't expect other people to accommodate your lifestyle. Some may be unaware, others may simply not know what to do and innocently prepare a dish they think you can eat. Understand that it's your responsibility, wherever you are, to stick to your gluten-free diet. You cannot, and shouldn't, rely on others.

What's For Dinner?

It is rude to tell your host or hostess that you can't eat the lasagna and that they should have something else for you. We repeat: don't expect special accommodations. However, it is perfectly acceptable to simply ask what they are serving.

Politely explain that the reason for your inquiry is that you have a dietary restriction. Perhaps the host will accommodate you; perhaps not. But knowing what you're getting yourself into will help you be prepared. You can eat before leaving for the event and then simply toy with a few vegetables without calling attention to yourself.

What if your host promised to prepare a gluten-free meal, but it turns out he or she has no idea what this entails and you end up with a fried chicken coated in flour? Again, it's a good idea to eat before arriving, despite the host's promises. Then, when you join the assembled guests, you can concentrate on having fun instead of focusing on the food. And don't pout at the host. He or she meant well but didn't know better than to serve anything breaded.

If you know the host well, or if it's family, ask if you can bring your own dish that will accommodate your diet. Very few people would take offense to such a request.

There will be times when neither you nor the host have enough control of the menu, such as when it's a large, catered affair. In such an event, don't even mention your diet. Fill up on healthy food before you arrive. There is every chance that such a function will have vegetables, salad, or a piece of meat that you can enjoy. If in doubt, quietly ask the catering staff.

As you go gluten-free, shift your socializing to having fun with people rather than focusing on the food.

You've Met Mr. or Ms. Right

Can you date and remain gluten-free? Of course, you can. It can be daunting until you get used to it, but if anyone makes a fuss, he or she deserves to be kicked to the curb, anyway.

Most first dates involve some type of food, so be upfront. Explain that your food options are limited due to health condition. How much you wish to elaborate is up to you.

Offer to help your date find an appropriate restaurant. ("Billy-Bob's All You Can Eat Pizza" probably won't make the list.) If he or she opts to make the selection, you should feel free to get the name of the restaurant beforehand. Call the restaurant before you go and ask them how they handle gluten-free recipes.

Most restaurants these days are willing to cooperate, but you want to make sure they don't cross-contaminate their ingredients. Ask how the food is prepared. These are not rude questions, and any restaurant that treats them as such shouldn't get your business.

If Mr. or Ms. Right makes light of your precautions, perhaps you should consider leaving them in the frog pond. Looking out for one's health is reasonable and smart.

At the restaurant, as you would in any social situation, concentrate on the other person and have fun. The focus should be to have a good time, not worrying about the food. But do feel free to ask the waiter any relevant questions.

You're the Host

Probably the best way to socialize and maintain control of your diet is for you to be the host. This will not only alleviate your worries, it's a great opportunity for you to educate your friends and family. When they ask about a dish they enjoy, tell them it is gluten-free.

This is likely to stimulate their interest and raise questions about the benefits of eating gluten-free. Use this time to enlighten and educate your friends. Who knows? You may make a few converts.

Finding a Restaurant

We have discussed calling restaurants and asking appropriate questions. Luckily, the number of gluten-free restaurants is on the rise. As for "regular" restaurants, your best bet is one with a large and diverse menu that will always have a simple steak and steamed veggies.

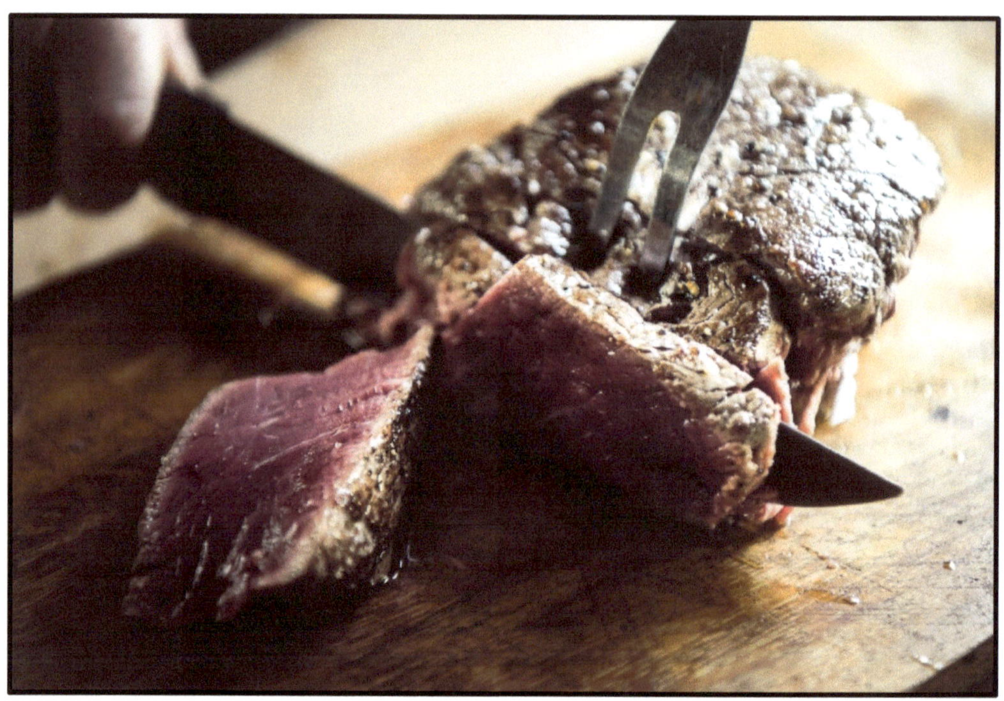

Certain types of restaurants are more likely to be safer for you than others.

1. BBQ restaurants are likely to focus on meat and potatoes. BBQ sauces are usually gluten-free, but don't hesitate to ask.

2. Don't discount fast food restaurants. The good thing about them is that they post the nutritional content of all of their food. Fries, a salad, or some chili should be safe to eat.

3. Oriental restaurants such as Indian, Thai, or Vietnamese have rice noodles as a standard part of their menu.

4. Steak and Seafood restaurants are another good bet. Meat, fish, potatoes and a vegetable can make an excellent gluten-free meal. Just stay away from anything breaded.

Make Gluten-Free Friends

If you join a gluten-free support group in your area, you will meet new people and make new friends that are in the same position as you. You will be surrounded by an entire group that is supportive and knowledgeable about gluten-free eating. That makes eating out and socializing a worry-free pleasure.

5

AVOIDING THE PITFALLS OF GLUTEN-FREE

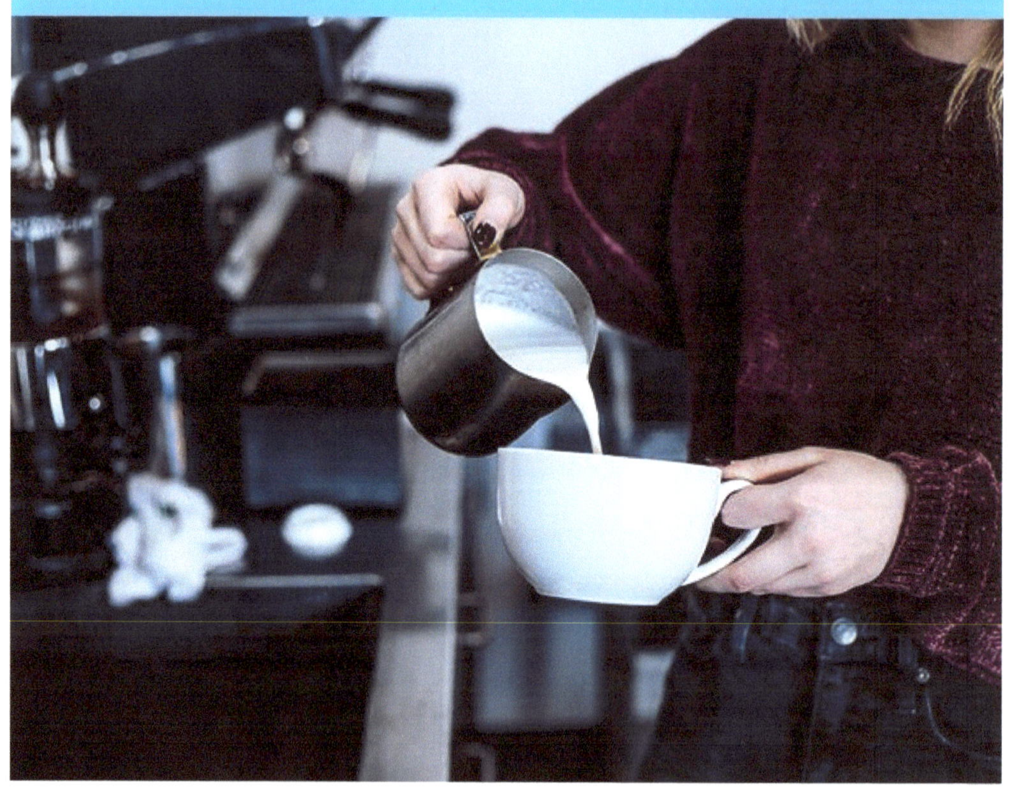

Chapter 5

Avoiding the Pitfalls of Gluten-Free

It's not just people with celiac disease that are opting for a gluten-free diet. According to the Mayo Clinic, 72 percent of people going gluten-free are doing so on the recommendation of a nutritionist or physician. Thankfully, the medical profession is no longer ignoring the fact that "new" processed wheat has nothing to offer us in terms of health and wellbeing and may be doing a variety of harm.

But jumping on the gluten-free bandwagon without enough facts can backfire. Unless you take the time to become informed, you are likely to continue feeling not as well as you could. The more you know about gluten, where it is and what it does, the better off you will be. The gluten-free life can be a challenge, and knowledge is your best ally. If your small intestine is damaged, even small mistakes can cause a setback and prevent recovery.

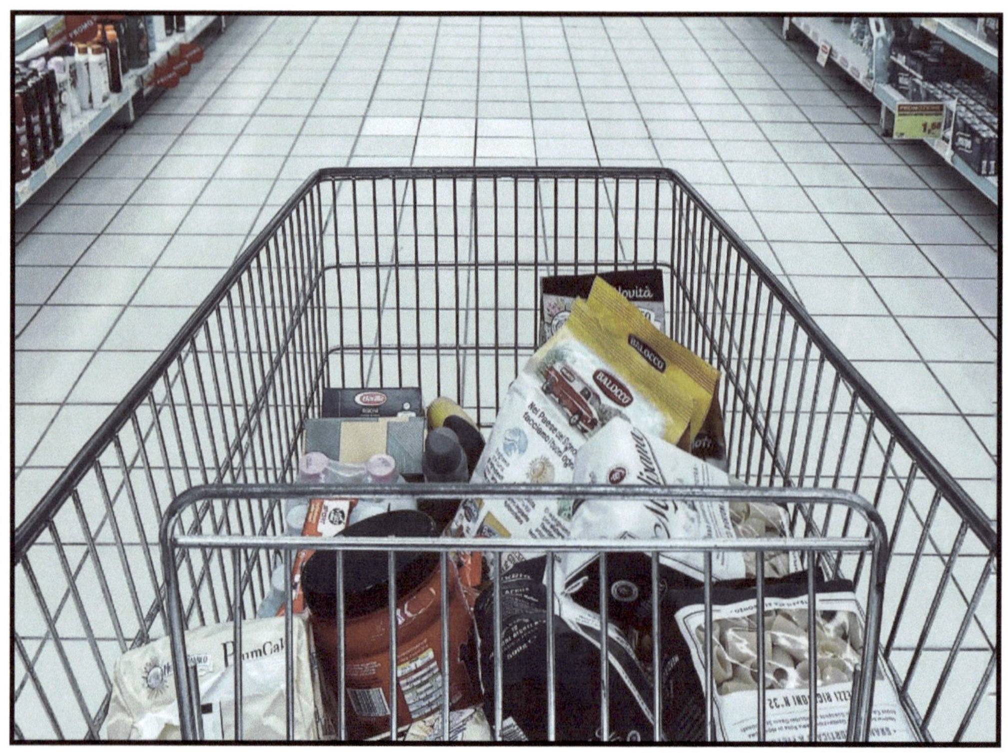

One of the major obstacles is that gluten can hide in the most unexpected places. Going gluten-free is not just a matter of abstaining from wheat products. Carefully read labels or ask questions, because gluten may find its way in the following food items:

1. Granola is hyped as a health food, but many of them are made of glutenous oats. Read the label first.

2. Certain types of potatoes chips have malt (wheat) vinegar in them.

3. Meat is gluten-free, but beware of processed meats such as deli meats, hot dogs, salami, and liverwurst, as they are processed with grain.

4. Canned soups can contain barley or wheat as a thickening agent. Again, read all labels.

5. Corn tortillas are usually gluten-free, but some add wheat.

6. Check all salad dressings and marinades.

7. Certain vegetarian "meats," such as vegetarian burgers, sausage or bacon, may contain gluten.

8. Some restaurants "puff" up their scrambled eggs with wheat batter. If in doubt, ask the waiter.

In addition to the hidden gluten, another problem with establishing a gluten-free diet is that you may not be getting all of the necessary nutrients. According to a study published in Clinical Nutrition, gluten-free eaters were likely to be deficient in vitamins D and B, zinc, magnesium, folate, iron and calcium.

The deficiency increases if non-glutenous bread, pasta, etc. are substituted for glutenous versions of these products. While gluten-free foods can be helpful and handy, many of them are processed with added sugars and fats, and they are not "fortified" with additional vitamins the way white flour foods frequently are.

Gluten-free versions of any food won't make you sick, but you should be very careful.

Ensuring a nutrient-dense life is not difficult at all. Increase vegetable and fruit servings to five a day and add quinoa and amaranth flour to your diet. The added fruits and vegetables will also provide you with the fiber you need.

To ensure that you get all your vitamins and minerals, eat plenty of the following foods:

1. Beas, peas, and legumes are an excellent source of thiamin.
2. Spinach and soybeans provide riboflavin
3. Avocado, chicken, broccoli, and salmon contain niacin.
4. Greens, spinach, asparagus, broccoli, and lettuce are a source of folate and magnesium.
5. For added iron, eat meat and lentils.
6. Seafood, especially salmon, provides Vitamin D.

Celiac disease, which can damage the small intestine, can make it difficult for the body to absorb all of the necessary nutrients. Discuss taking a supplement with your doctor or pharmacist. To get all possible nutrients from the food you eat, increase your intake of raw fruits and vegetables as opposed to cooking them. Choose a wide variety of produce that include as many colors as possible.

Another reason you may not be seeing the hoped-for progress on your gluten-free diet is that the damage to the small intestine is so severe, even permitted grains such as rice or corn may continue to be a problem. Nuts, while gluten-free, are also difficult to digest. If you continue to experience gastrointestinal problems, check with your doctor.

You may wish to wait until your small intestine has recovered sufficiently before enjoying those food items. Try to abstain from all grains and nuts, even the permitted kinds, until your small intestine is back on track. This may take a while, so be patient. You want the intestine to heal, don't you?

In addition, while gluten-free products can be helpful, too many companies are jumping on the gluten-free trend. Many of these products are over-processed and filled with sugars and fats and may come close to resembling any other processed food item. A better solution is to invest in a few reputable gluten-free cookbooks and prepare your meals from scratch.

Traveling Gluten-Free

You don't want additional drama while traveling, but how are you supposed to control your diet while on the road? Many people on a gluten-free diet unravel their eating habits due to poor planning. As always, preparation is the key to success.

If you are driving, it's best to avoid those roadside eateries. Simply pack a cooler with sandwiches on gluten-free bread. For snacks and for the kids, make sure you have plenty of nuts, cheese, fruits (including dried fruits), and gluten-free crackers. Pack the same foods for flight travel and long waits at the airport. You can purchase most kinds of potato chips safely (exempt malt vinegar-flavored) at any airport newsstand.

Do some research for any gluten-free restaurants along your travel route.

EMOTIONAL OBSTACLES TO HAVING CELIAC DISEASE

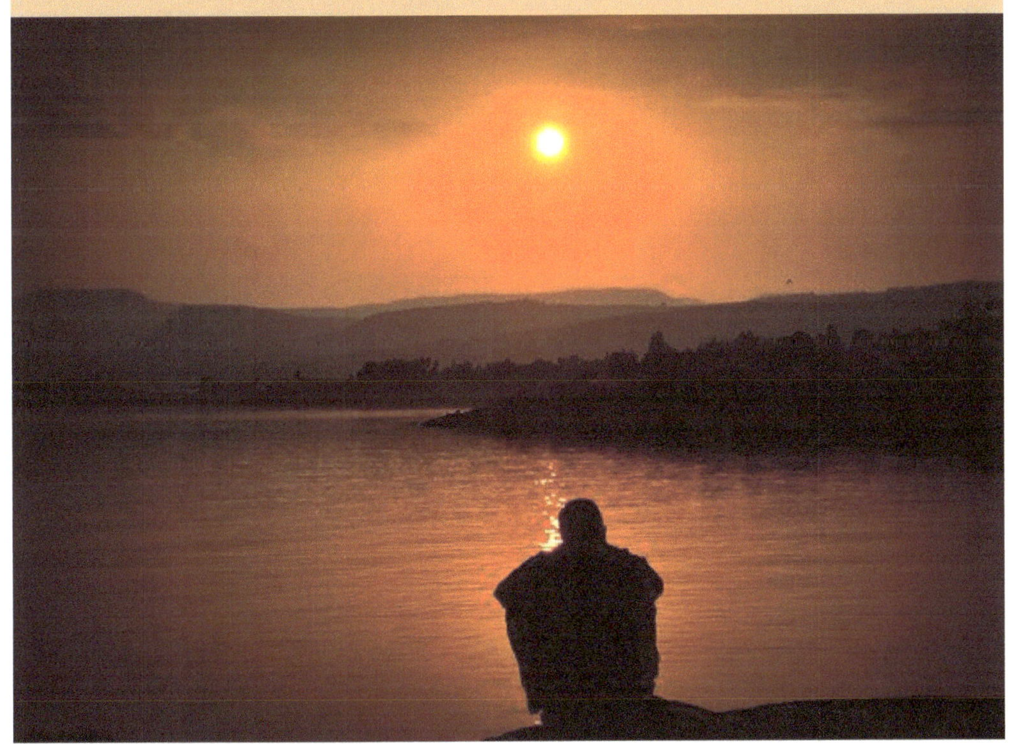

Chapter 6

Emotional Obstacles to Having Celiac Disease

A diagnosis of celiac disease can seem overwhelming. It's perfectly okay to feel upset. Celiac disease is serious, and it needs to be handled. You will undoubtedly feel shock at the diagnosis. Your first reaction may be denial.

This can't be happening to you! All you can feel is a crushing frustration and anger at the unfairness of it all. These are perfectly normal reactions. There is no reason for you to deny your emotions. Feel whatever you need to feel. After all, this diagnosis will change a large part of your life.

At some point, you need to reach acceptance. You've been feeling sick and miserable for so long, you want to feel better. This is your chance. So, it up to you to become determined and deal with the situation.

Make no mistake. This may not be easy, especially if the decision to go gluten-free isn't your own. Here is why celiac disease can be such a difficult diagnosis to accept:

1. So many of our social interactions revolve around food. You have every right to wonder how this will change once you go gluten-free.

2. Family and friends may not understand your situation. Perhaps some of them tell you to just get over yourself. You may be accused of having an eating disorder. "It's just toast and scrambled eggs. Eat, for heaven sakes!" This lack of support just makes a difficult situation harder.

3. Knowing you'll need to give up some of your favorite can produce understandable anxiety. There is truth in the term "comfort food." Certain foods do comfort us. After your diagnosis, you realize your options will be limited. You have certain favorite dishes that you may not be able to enjoy anymore. It feels like losing a friend.

4. You will need to make some changes in your life. Depending on how well you react to change, that, too, can bring on anxiety.

5. You will have to follow new rules, and that isn't always easy. You used to be in control of your eating habits. Now you have to follow someone's rules!

6. There is no known cure for celiac disease. All you can do is alleviate the symptoms by changing your eating habits. Yes, celiac is something you'll have to live with forever.

7. Everyone around you is munching on Oreo cookies and devouring hamburger buns. You feel alone and isolated.

8. A major problem for celiac sufferers is that they develop a gluten-free lifestyle, stick to it, and feel so much better after a while. That's when the rumbling in the brain can start. "I'm fine now. I can have that slice of pizza or cookie." "Grandma prepared this especially for me. I have to eat it." This can be one of the most difficult periods you'll have to with. You're so tempted … just one slice.

It's crucial to resist temptation. You're feeling better because you've eliminated gluten from your diet. Remember how miserable you felt before your new diet. Don't reverse the course that will force you to start over. You're exactly where you want to be. Keep going.

When You Are Tempted to Cheat

Sometimes, the urge to cheat – just a little bit – can be overwhelming. This is especially true when special occasions arise. So many of our holiday memories are tied to food.

The problem is, there is no such thing as cheating "a little" when you have celiac disease. Even a minuscule amount of gluten can affect the immune system. So, it's not a matter of just one bite." For someone with celiac disease, any bite is a bite too many. Even people who are "only" gluten-sensitive can be severely affected by a small amount of it.

Gluten may cause the gut to leak from the small intestine, which can cause toxins to spread into the body and cause inflammations.

Consider seriously if mom's delicious stack of pancakes is worth this. This book is intended to help you make good choices.

The most serious case of cheating is done by gluten-sensitive people who don't show immediate negative symptoms. They may continue cheating, and gut is being damaged, although they don't know it until their autoimmune system is adversely affected. If you have been exposed to gluten, get a lab test before the damage caused become irreversible.

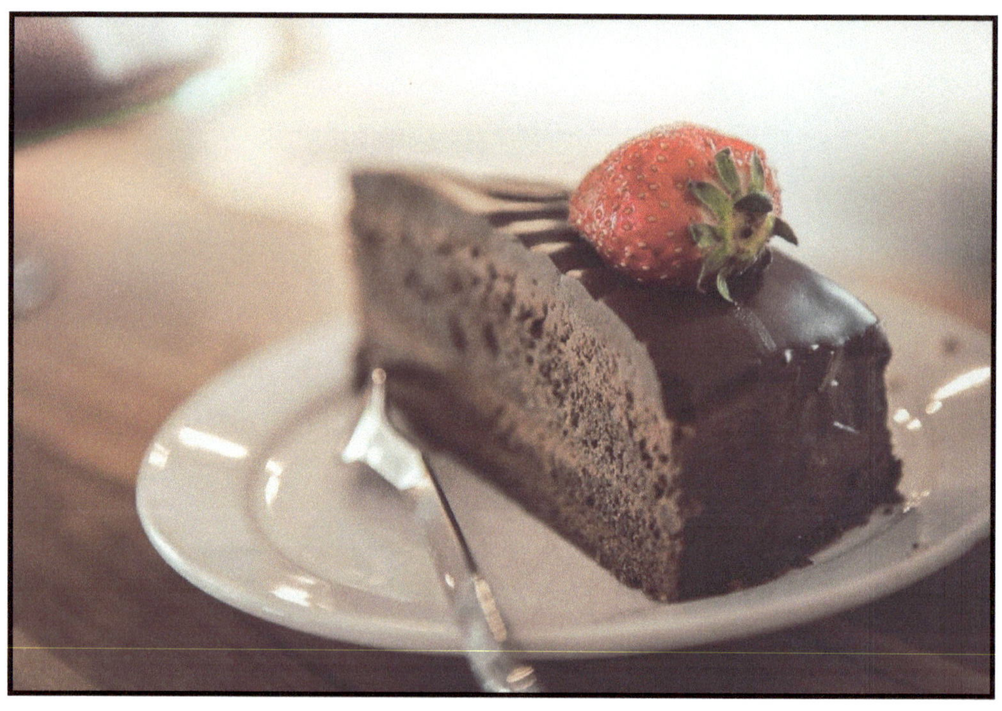

Cravings can pop up at any time. They can be difficult to handle, but you are in control. Like an alcoholic, take it one day at a time. You may want that piece of cake more than life itself at this moment. Just get through the moment. Walk away, if possible. Understand that the craving won't be as severe the next day. We repeat: handle cravings one day at a time and remain in control.

You also need to understand what foods trigger your cravings. Is it going to mom's house and having her prepare all of your childhood favorites? Is going out with friends for pizza too difficult to handle?

If you can't avoid the triggers (you really can't avoid mom), learn to handle them. Talk to mom about celiac disease and how to prepare gluten-free options; or bring your own. Discover pizza parlors with gluten-free selections and convince your friends to go there. Remember, cheating is always a choice. Make good choices for yourself.

Taking Control of Your Emotions

Let's not fool ourselves. Knowing you are suffering from celiac disease can cause bouts of blues and depression. When you start feeling down, it's time to elevate your emotions instead of obsessing on food. Following are some ways to feel better and enjoy a higher quality of life.

1. Depression can make you withdraw, but you need to reach out. Have at least one person you can talk to about what you are going through without worrying about judgments being made. This can be a parent, sibling, best friend, someone else who has celiac disease, or a professional. Just feeling understood can lift your spirits tremendously.

2. Instead of withdrawing, become *more* involved with people. Reach out to someone who is going through a rough time. Find a worthwhile association where you can volunteer and make a difference. Everyone is dealing with *something*. Knowing that will make you feel less alone.

3. While a pet won't replace other people, it can help you feel less alone.

4. Discover a new hobby or interest to get your mind off food. Taking a class, joining a gym, becoming involved in your community can be very energizing. Life has too much to offer to make it all about food.

5. If certain people are unsupportive of your situation or perhaps actually accusing you of overreacting, consider whether these people should remain in your life? What exactly are they adding to it?

6. Remove as much stress from your life as possible. Consider practicing meditation for half an hour daily. Just find a comfortable seat, close your eyes, and focus on your breath as you inhale and exhale. This will relax your mind and spirit.

7. Nature seems to be the best medicine of all. If you live in a city, find a park and walk around, enjoying what nature has to offer. Take a walk during your lunch hour. If you live in the country, communing with nature is even easier. It is true that sunshine will boost your day.

7

GLUTEN, ADHD AND AUTISM

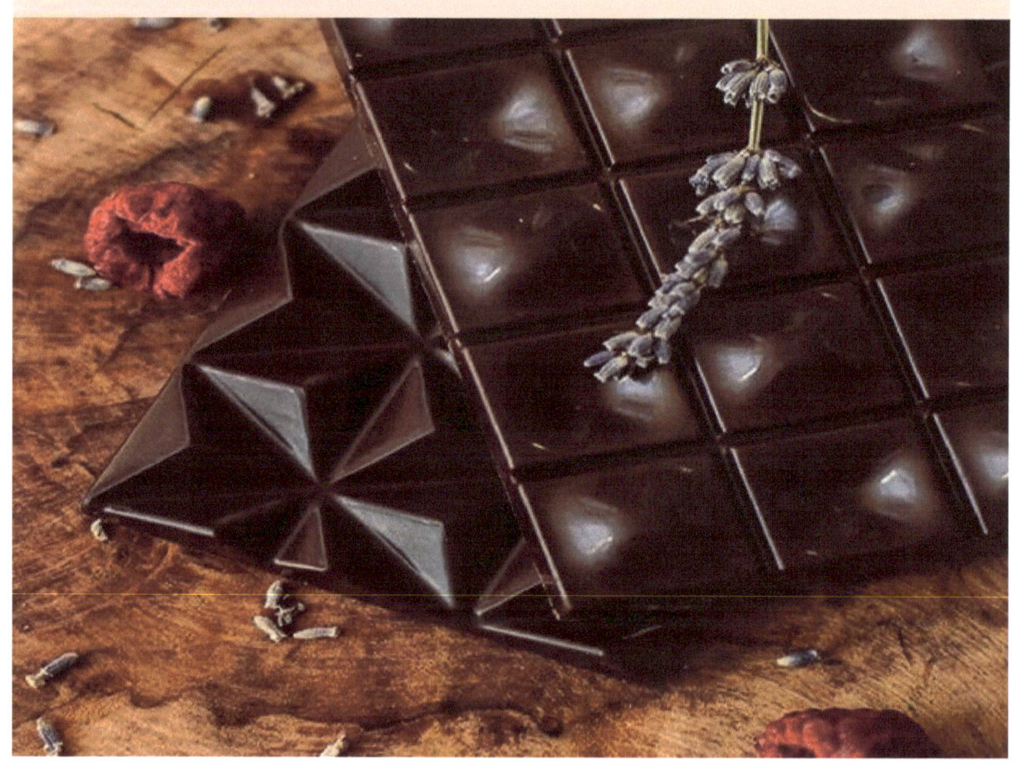

Chapter 7

Gluten, ADHD and Autism

ADHD – attention deficit hyperactivity disorder – is on the rise. It is difficult to diagnose (and treat), but as the name implies, it involves the amount of hyperactivity in children. The connection between celiac disease and ADHD is still being studied, but doctors and parents have noticed that both are connected to food allergies and/or food intolerance. Interestingly, around 70 percent of ADHD sufferers have a sensitivity to gluten.

We know that the frontal brain lobe, which is in charge of memory and planning activity is impaired in people with ADHD. It is also known that gluten can affect that very area of the brain. Therefore, more and more researchers and doctors are treating ADHD by omitting gluten from the diet.

Kids with ADHD react differently when gluten is removed from their diet. But the results have been quite incredible. The kids have become less hyperactive and decreased mental confusion. In each study, the researchers found that giving up gluten resulted in improved brain function in all cases.

When the connection between autism and gluten was studied, two-thirds of the children showed improvement once they were no longer eating gluten. They are still working to connect the two factors, but the results have astounded them. They cannot be denied.

One of the challenges for parents, of course, is picky little eaters. Some children are extremely adamant in what they will eat and what they won't go near. They may only eat one kind of food or even food of one color. Kids with ADHD may also react negatively to sugar, so parents need to remove both from their diet.

In a 2006 study, 132 participants were tested for celiac disease and ADHD. Subsequently, the participants were given a diet free of gluten for six months. When the researchers checked them after that time period, they found that many participants with undiagnosed celiac disease also had ADHD. They concluded that a diet free of gluten could benefit these participants.

Both people suffering from celiac disease and ADHD show man.

Celiac disease sufferers complain of many similar discomforts: symptoms as ADHD sufferers do. This may include headaches, difficulty in focusing, abdominal pain and others. Researchers have notice such an overlap in symptoms that some believe that anyone tested for celiac disease should automatically be screened for ADHD.

Of course, not all people with ADHD suffer from celiac disease but may still benefit from a gluten-free diet. The reason is that a gluten-free diet, when properly adhered to, should be more nutrient-dense than the average diet. This means that someone with ADHD on a gluten-free diet will be eating less processed foods and consume more healthy meats, fish, and produce and see symptoms improve as a result.

All-to-frequently, when kids with ADHD go to school, the gluten-free diet is given up as unsustainable. These kids find it difficult to sit still for lengthy periods of time. This forces them back on medication. A number of parents have solved the problems by reinstituting a gluten-free diet (yes, it's hard to control kids when they are in school). Parents have found that the kids improved enough to have their medication lowered considerably.

Gluten-Free and Autism

So far, there has been too little research on autism and gluten-free diets. Autism is a disorder of the brain which can make it difficult for a child to communicate and socialize.

Stony Brook University researchers studied 59 children diagnosed with autism and 44 of their non-autistic siblings. The children's family were to record all of their food intake and take stool samples.

The researchers found that almost half of the autistic children, and 30 percent of the non-autistic siblings, suffered from gastrointestinal disorder. These numbers are much higher than found in the general population of children. Since gastrointestinal issues involved the small intestine, researchers have concluded that a gluten-free diet may prove beneficial.

If your child suffers from AHDH or autism, discuss the possibility of a gluten-free diet with his or her pediatrician. While more studies need to be conducted, placing your child on a healthy gluten-free diet won't hurt him or her, and it might help. Be sure to discuss any specific dietary changes with your child's doctor.

Beware of Chocolate

Kids love chocolate, and you don't want to deprive them. The good news is, you and the kids don't have to give up your favorite sweet on your gluten-free diet. You just have to pick the right chocolate bar. Some are gluten-free, others aren't.

The problem isn't chocolate, as the cacao bean is naturally gluten-free. However, most candy bars add a number of ingredients, and that's what you need to watch out for. A rule of thumb is that the more ingredients in a chocolate bar, the greater the chances there will be a wheat by-product.

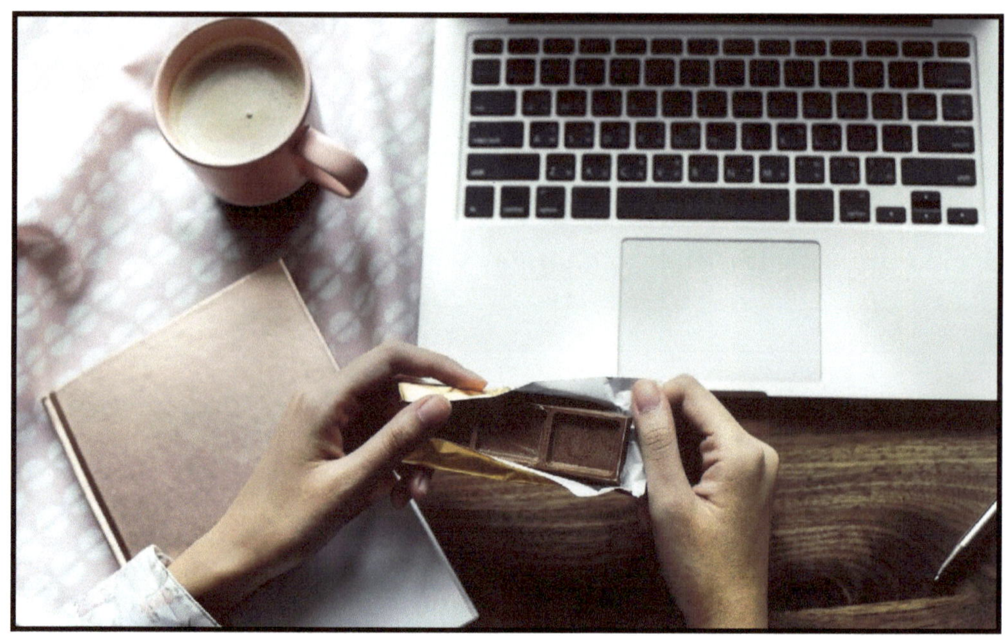

Chocolate bars that contain a cookie are off-limits. Malt balls are made with malt and contain gluten.

Milk chocolates such as Hershey's Milk Chocolate Bar is made with milk and is gluten-free.

When it comes to white chocolate, you need to read the labels. Generally, white chocolate is made with sugar and shea butter and is gluten-free. But that does not apply to every brand of white chocolate. Lindt's white chocolate contains gluten, while Ghirardelli's White Chocolate baking bar does not.

While many chocolate manufacturers make gluten-free chocolate, they use the same equipment to manufacture their gluten chocolates without cleaning the machines, thereby risking cross-contamination.

Chocolate-lovers can relax, however. There are a number of safe, gluten-free chocolates on the market:

- Alter Eco – almost all of their premium chocolates are gluten-free.
- Nestlé Milk Chocolate is gluten-free
- Dove Chocolate – these chocolates contain no gluten.
- Enjoy Life chocolate – These chocolate bars are manufactured on gluten-free equipment and are totally gluten-free.
- Hershey's – The famous Hershey Kisses and the Hershey milk chocolate are gluten-free. Their other candies may contain gluten.
- Scharffen Berger Chocolate makes both dark and milk chocolate bars that are gluten-free.
- Vosges Haut Chocolate makes chocolates with some interesting flavors, most of which are gluten-free. Check the label.

To keep your child from being tempted by chocolate when among friends, tuck a few satisfying Hershey's Kisses in his or her bag.

ADAPTING YOUR DIET TO GLUTEN-FREE

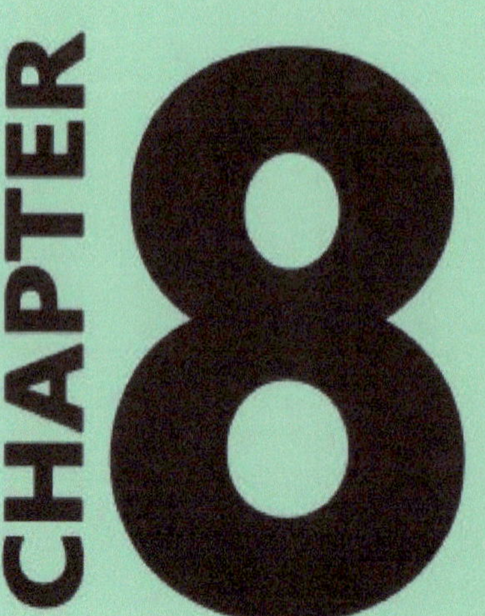

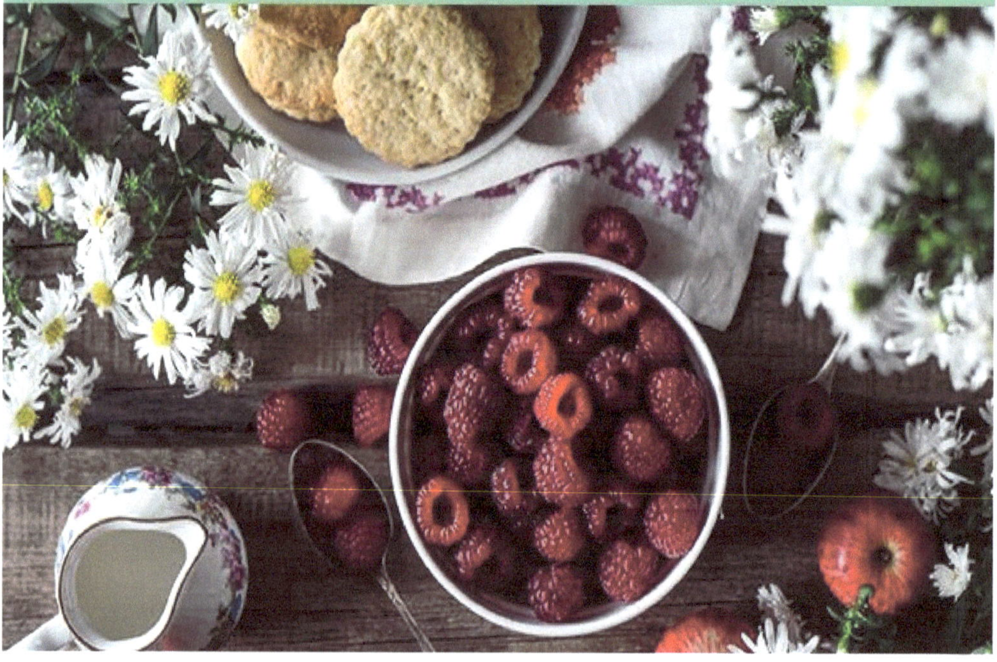

Chapter 8

Adapting Your Diet to Gluten-Free

Once you go gluten-free, you can still enjoy the same dishes you've always loved. As already stated, you aren't giving up anything; you are adding better health to your life. You just need to get creative about preparation techniques. Keep in mind that just about *any* dish can be made gluten-free.

Baking Your Favorite Treats the Gluten-Free Way

We promised at the beginning of this book that you could savor your favorite cookies, pies, and cakes on a gluten-free diet. Using gluten-free flours can be challenging, but it's still possible to create tasty goodies for yourself and your family. Here are some tips for changing your gluten-sweets into gluten-free:

1. When using gluten-free flour, increase the baking powder and baking soda by a quarter. If a standard recipe calls for a teaspoon of baking soda, use a teaspoon and a quarter.

2. Gluten-free flour can crumble. Therefore, making smaller versions of your usual cookies, or baking individual pies instead of one large one, will help keep everything stuck together. When baking breads, bake two mini-loaves instead of a single loaf.

3. Improve the quality and taste of baked goods by combining various types of gluten-free flour instead of using just one kind.

4. Use starches for added texture when you bake. Every recipe can differ, so you need to experiment. A good guide is to use 3 cups of flour to ½ cup of starch. Starch can be tapioca, potato starch, or cornstarch. It bears repeating that baking is not a precise science, and you may need to experiment a few times with the ratio for the perfect combination.

5. Gluten is what helps a dough stick together. Without gluten, you need to use something else to keep your dish from falling apart. Use a teaspoon or more of guar gum, gelatin, or xanthan to keep

your breads together. For cakes and muffins, add only half a teaspoon. Adding an extra egg can also help bind the dry ingredients together.

6. Yes, you are likely to make mistakes when you experiment. But you don't have to let everything go to waste. Place those errors in a food processor and create gluten-free coating for your fried meats and fish.

7. To create a more perfect gluten-free dough, beat the batter more than you would ordinary dough to provide it with some structure.

8. Butter is a permitted addition to your gluten-free baking. However, to add extra sweetness, moisture, and nutrition, substitute a portion of the butter called for with a fruit puree. The best fruits to use are apples, avocados, and bananas. They can add a great deal of flavor to baked goods.

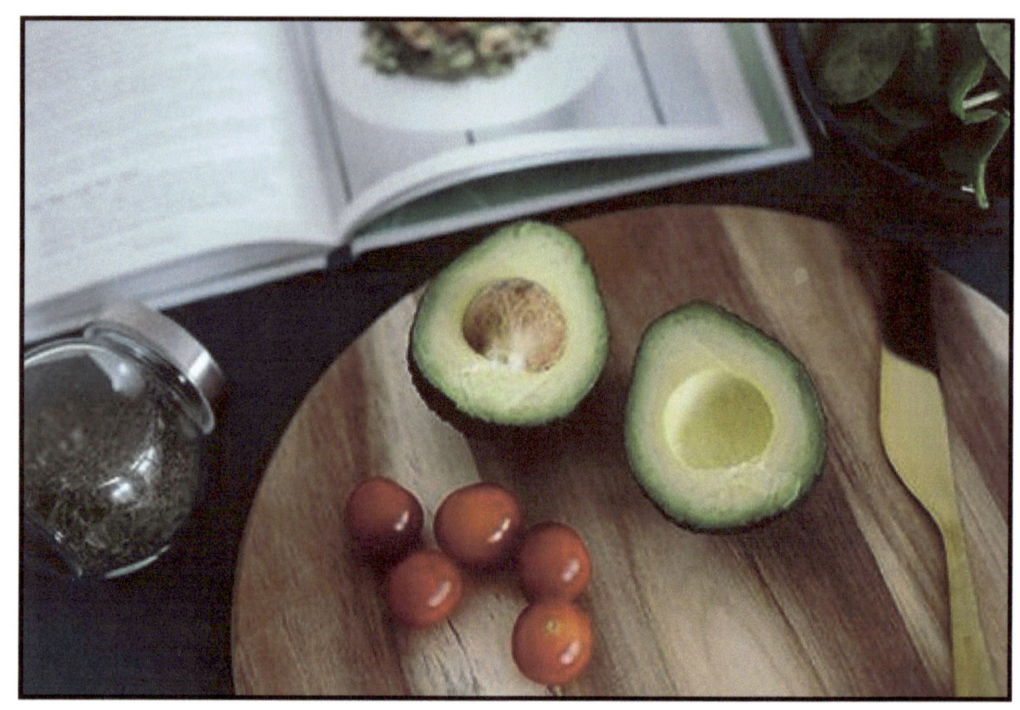

Making Good Substitutions in Your Recipes

Get creative when cooking gluten-free and learn how to multi-use your ingredients:

1. Anything that calls for a bun can be wrapped in lettuce or a corn tortilla.

2. You don't have to give up your favorite fried chicken, pork chops, or fish. Just substitute a different coating for the usual breadcrumbs. We have already discussed turning some failed baking attempts into crumbs. You can also turn gluten-free

bread into breadcrumbs. Another interesting way to coat is to crumble up pork rinds.

3. Some recipes call for beer. Unless you have a non-malt, gluten-free beer handy, use apple cider instead.

4. To make croutons for your salads, cut up a few slices of gluten-free bread and fry the cubes.

5. When preparing sandwiches, don't limit yourself to gluten-free bread. Get creative and use corn tortillas, waffles, or thin pancakes. Also, try a healthful lettuce wrap.

Mastering gluten-free cooking takes some creativity and experimentation. It's a good idea to try smaller batches until you achieve satisfying results.

Being diagnosed with celiac disease or wheat allergy does not have to interfere with your favorite meals. Play around with the ingredients and enjoy tasty results.

Conclusion

Receiving a diagnosis of celiac disease or gluten intolerance can be a shock that can come out of the blue. Even if you've made your own decision to abstain from eating gluten for reasons of health, you may feel somewhat overwhelmed. You know changes are necessary, but how do you even get started?

Understand that giving up some of your favorite food items is a loss, especially when you didn't expect it. Allow yourself time to feel that loss.

1. You want to deny what the doctor is telling you. He or she can't possibly be correct. Doctors make mistakes all the time. While you're in denial, however, you feel tired, uncomfortable, and continue reacting badly to wheat.

2. You become angry. Who is someone to tell you that you can't go to your favorite pizza place!

3. After you deal with the anger, you mentally try to bargain with yourself. OK, so I may have celiac disease. But eating just one piece of cake at the party can't possibly hurt.

4. When the truth sinks in, you are likely to feel depressed. My life is over!

5. It may take a while, but acceptance finally sets in. You do some research and realize you can still eat what you want and do what you have always done. The only real change in your life will be that you begin to feel so much better than you have in the past.

When you have shifted your mindset, you are ready to begin going gluten-free. Once you understand the health benefits of giving up that unrefined flour, it is doubtful you will be seriously tempted to go back to the old, glutenous ways of eating. Going gluten-free is a lifetime commitment.

- Do some research and learn how wheat has changed from a life-sustaining food staple to a mangled grain that many people cannot process. The gluten in grain is actually making people sick.

- Rid your home of all gluten. Clean out the pantry, refrigerator and check the bathroom cabinets for any items containing gluten. Clean your pots, pans, and utensils to ensure that no cross-contamination occurs. Gluten can attach itself to many items in your home.

- Learning how to navigate the supermarket aisles when shopping will help you stock up on fresh, healthy food items and avoid dangerous temptations. It's important to always have a few staples on hand for quick meals and snacks. This will keep you from reaching for something that can ultimately make you ill. Plan your meals before you shop to make sure you have the necessary ingredients on hand.

- Just because you are eliminating gluten from your diet doesn't mean you can't continue socializing and eating out with friends and family. Many restaurants these days are able to accommodate a gluten-free diet. Check out local eateries and ask about their food preparation process.

  When dining at the home of friends and family, don't expect them to change their eating habits for you. They may try, but they may not know what to do. If in doubt, eat something healthful before visiting and concentrate on enjoying the company. Don't hesitate to discuss your dietary limitations when the subject arises.

- If you begin a gluten-free diet without knowing exactly what the diet entails, you could be undercutting your efforts. It's not just about eliminating breads, cookies, and cakes. Gluten can lurk in many foods, so learn to read labels with great care. Make sure your diet isn't nutrient-deprived by eating plenty of fresh produce each day. Eat a wide variety of foods to enjoy the best possible nutritional advantage.

- Even as you feel better and more energetic, you may still have moments of feeling deprived. That is perfectly normal. Learn daily habits that let you deal successfully with negative emotions. Adding exercise and new activities to your routine will expand your lifestyle and keep you from focusing only on food.

- Many interesting studies are being done with gluten and children with ADHD and autism. Much more research is needed, but a number of tests have shown that removing gluten from the diet of children suffering from ADHD or autism has had an extremely beneficial effect. This is something that should be discussed with your child's pediatrician.

- Baking, which always entails using flour, can be the biggest gluten-free challenge. Learn about all the substitutions you can make to prepare your old favorite treats and the best cooking techniques for gluten-free baking. You will be pleasantly surprised.

Celiac disease and wheat allergies are painful. If you are gluten-sensitive, there is no reason for you to feel miserable. Take the necessary steps to rid your life of gluten and start enjoying each day again. This could be one of the most important health decisions you will ever make.